Lose 40 Pounds
In 5 Months
Without Exercise

Kimberly E. Hanke

Large Print

Copyright November 30, 2017, by Kimberly E. Hanke

No portion of this booklet may be reproduced in any form without the express written permission of the author.

I want to thank numerous family and friends who offered their encouragement throughout these months of dieting and writing this booklet.

I would like to thank the makers of the following brand-name products suggested in this diet plan:

Vita Lea, OSTEOMATRIX, and Energizing Soy Protein are all trademarks and brands of the Shaklee Corporation, Pleasanton, CA 94588.

Premier Protein is a trademark and brand of the Premier Nutrition Corporation, Emeryville, CA, 94608.

Otter Pops is a trademark and brand of The Jel Sert Company, West Chicago, IL, 60186.

Metamucil is a trademark and brand of the Proctor & Gamble Company, Cincinnati, OH, 45202.

Lipton iced tea is a trademark and brand of Unilever, Englewood Cliffs, NJ, 07632.

Stevia Extract is a trademark and brand of Safeway Inc., Pleasanton, CA, 94588.

I was not compensated by any of the above companies for promoting their products in this booklet.

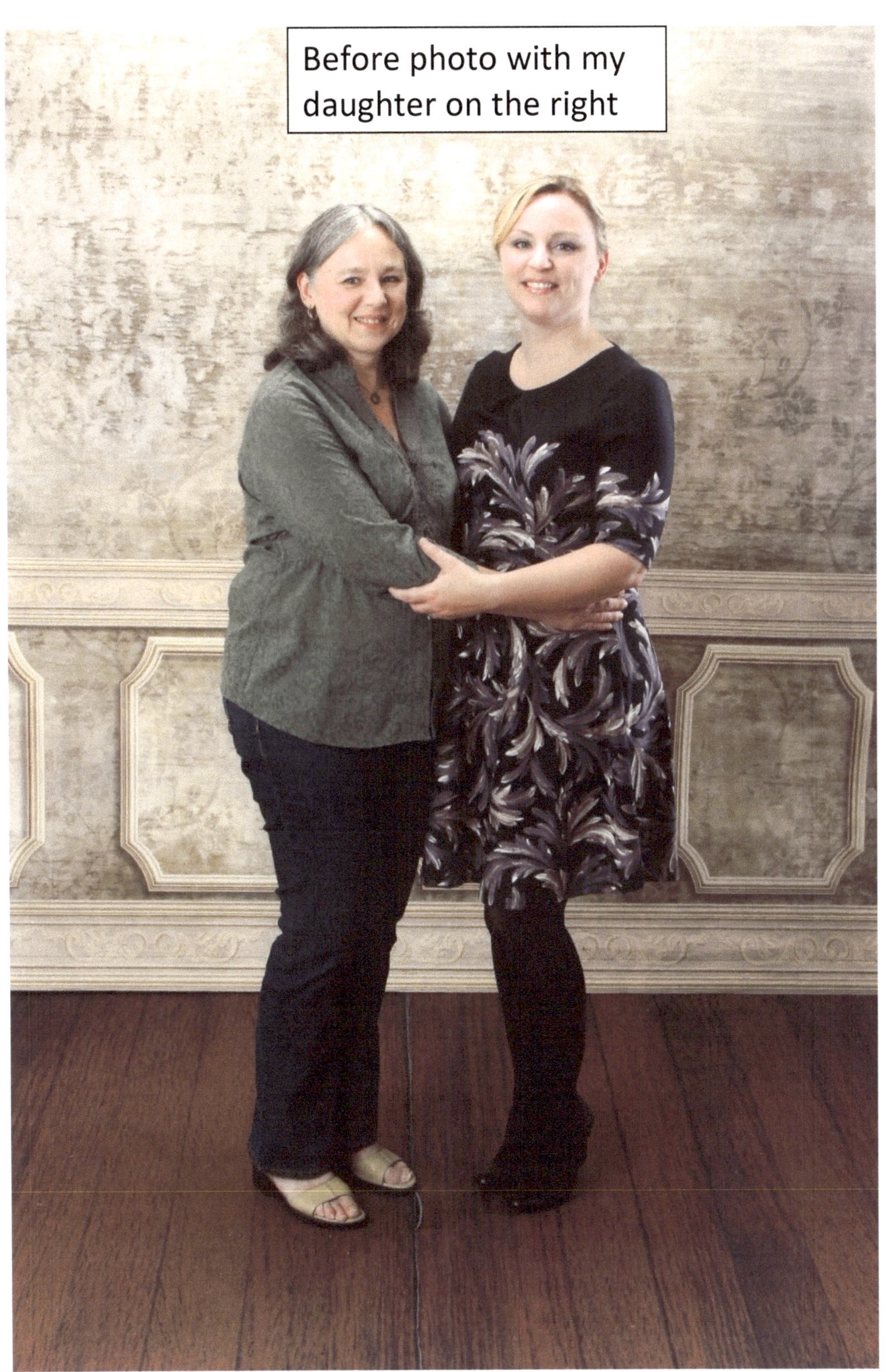

Before photo with my
daughter on the right

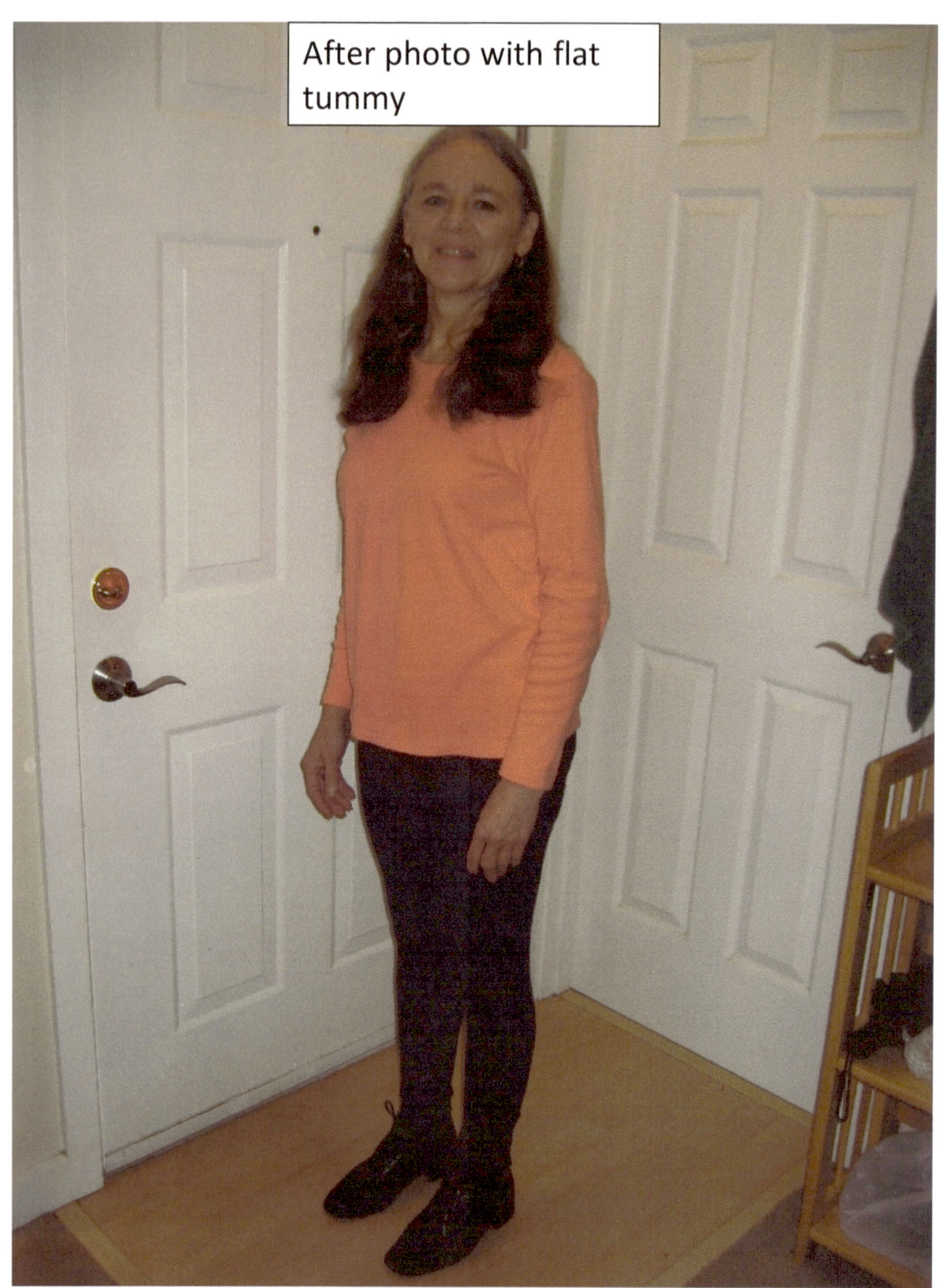

After photo with flat
tummy

Introduction

When I saw the "before" photo, I realized I had become overweight - the heaviest ever in my life. It wasn't until shopping in a plus size store that I made the decision I didn't want to fit into those clothes. Also, I didn't want to become another victim of Type 2 Diabetes. It was time to take charge of my body. If you do nothing, you get nothing.

Nutrition was important to me so I began by looking up the nutritional content of foods online. I chose foods that were highest in nutrition and lowest in calories. Nutrition is the key element to this diet.

I realized that food supplements were going to be necessary if I was going to get all the protein, fiber, and other nutrients I would need to get into my low calorie diet.

Other than nutritional supplements, I took no pills, specifically no diet pills. I wanted a diet that I could live with for a long period of time.

At that time, I didn't know that I would be having surgery on my foot and therefore be incapable of exercising for three months.

My original aim was for 1,200 calories per day but once the foods were analyzed and chosen, they added up to only 980 calories per day.

I was not in a hurry to lose the weight. Slow and steady works better long term and makes it easier to keep the weight off after reaching your optimal weight.

See the Preparation Time section to see how I eased into this diet. It took me two months to prepare myself before I was ready to commit to this diet in earnest.

By June first I was ready to begin.

This diet worked for me. I began in June at 174 pounds and lost 40 pounds by the end of October. I assume this will work for most adult women as I had this success when I was 61 years old.

Every day I successfully stayed on the diet was an accomplishment. The longer I chose to stick with it, the better I felt about myself. You can too. Every month, when I got on the scale, I was ecstatic to realize I had lost more pounds!

Friends told me they were amazed that I continued losing weight without any exercise. I did not exercise the entire time I was on this diet. I'm not particularly proud of that but it proved to me that I could lose the weight by diet alone. Of course, your general health will benefit and your weight loss will increase if you do exercise.

This plan was created by and for me, to ensure I got all the necessary nutrition while adhering to this low calorie diet. I am sharing it because I had great success and realized that others could benefit from this diet plan, too.

I am not an expert in the field of nutrition, but like you, I can read nutrition labels and check the RDA (recommended daily allowance for nutrients). I suggest you bring this booklet to your doctor to find out if you need to make any adjustments to this diet due to your gender and your particular health conditions. Also ask your doctor what is your optimal weight. This will be your goal.

This diet is based on taking in 1,000 calories per day while getting necessary nutrition, including enough protein and fiber. This has worked for me and it is important for me, personally, to supplement calcium so I take more than this diet plan suggests.

Percentage of RDA is based on a 2,000 calorie diet. However, calorie needs and subsequent nutritional percent of RDA differs based on gender, age, and level of activity.

My calculations rely on the nutrition labels of the brand-named products included here. For items without a brand name, I looked up their nutrition and calories online on numerous websites.

Read through this entire booklet at least once before you begin preparations or begin the diet itself.

% of RDA - Daily Nutrition Totals of this Diet Plan:

Calories   980 calories per day

Protein   59 grams or 118% of recommended daily

                allowance for protein

Fiber   41 grams or 164% of RDA

Sodium   963 mg or 64% of RDA, making this a low sodium

                diet (less than 1,500 mg)

Calcium   174% of RDA or 1,744 mg

Vitamin A   216% of RDA

Vitamin C   720% of RDA

Vitamin D3   200% of RDA or 800 IU (from Vita Lea alone)

Vitamin E   228% of RDA

Vitamin K   181% of RDA

Thiamin   264% of RDA

Riboflavin   250% of RDA

Niacin   179% of RDA

Vitamin B6   161% of RDA

Folate   139% of RDA

Vitamin B12   125% of RDA

Biotin   125% of RDA

Pantothenic Acid   150% of RDA

Phosphorus   115% of RDA

Iodine   125% of RDA

Magnesium   138% of RDA

Zinc   132% of RDA

Selenium   125% of RDA

Copper   86% of RDA

Manganese   134% of RDA

Molybdenum   125% of RDA

Iron   71% of RDA if taking Vita Lea without iron. Vita Lea with iron adds 100% more iron.

Potassium   83% of RDA

Preparation Time - One Month Minimum
(It took me two months)

You need to give yourself time to gradually make some changes that would be difficult to make all at once when you start this diet. If you make substitutions to items I list, compare their nutrition labels and calorie counts to the brand names listed in this booklet. The following are examples of the preparations I made before starting this diet.

- Drink more water.

- Brush your teeth after meals to clear your mouth of any food taste.

- Practice saying no. Say no to one candy bar or one soda at a time. Saying no gets easier with continual practice.

- If you are craving chocolate, buy one small piece of chocolate at the checkout counter instead of a regular candy bar.

- If you want cake, pie, or a brownie, buy one piece instead of an entire cake, pie, or batch of brownies.

- Don't buy a regular bag of potato chips; buy a small bag.

- Buy a scoop of ice cream, not a half gallon carton. It's worth the extra money.

- Give yourself constant encouragement. Imagine you are talking to a good friend and speak just as kindly to yourself. Every day.

- Take charge of your stress and anxiety levels. Stress and anxiety may cause food cravings. Do whatever you can to simplify your life, make peace with others, and make an effort to relax.

- Set your alarm 30 minutes earlier, causing you less stress in the morning. Leave for work 15 minutes earlier so you won't stress as much about your commute.

- Change what you need to so that you can sleep 8 hours each night.

- Taper off and then stop drinking sodas of any kind

- If you want a flavored drink, try iced tea with Stevia sweetener.

- If you put sugar in your coffee or tea, use Stevia sweetener instead of sugar; it has no calories.

- Eat smaller portions to get your stomach used to less food.

- Don't eat over the sink. Sit down for your meals.

- Eat slower. Give yourself time to enjoy the food you are eating. Take smaller bites. This will also help you notice when you've had enough.

- Eat until you are satisfied instead of eating until you are full. This is crucial.

- Eat breakfast within an hour of getting up in the morning. This jumpstarts your metabolism for the day. Don't skip it.

- Don't skip meals at all. This is part of learning to have a healthier attitude toward food.

- Remind yourself of your best reasons to lose the weight. Maybe your best reason is to get rid of Type 2 Diabetes. Perhaps your best reason is to fit into clothes you want. Or maybe you are tired of feeling embarrassed about your weight. What are your most compelling reasons to lose the weight? Write them down.

- Fill your refrigerator with fruits and vegetables. Experiment with eating them raw or cooking them. Don't add butter or margarine. Add spices for flavor.

- Gradually eliminate high calorie snacks and treats; substitute with low calorie popsicles - no more than fifty calories each.

- Getting hungry an hour before a meal is normal and healthy. Drink water to hold you over. Also, you may be a little hungry at bedtime. That is okay; it's not time to eat.

- Clean out your cupboards and refrigerator. Remove all high calorie foods and treats.

- If you live with others, keep your food in a separate cupboard. Begin to gradually introduce your family to lighter fare instead of high calorie and high fat foods. This will help you transition into the diet, your transition when you reach your weight goal, and contribute to the health of your family.

- Begin adding some of this diet's ingredients into your daily diet. Start by taking two Vita Lea tablets each day to supplement the nutrition you're currently getting.

- Most importantly, commit to getting yourself healthy. You skip high calorie treats because they contain almost no nutritional value. You add fresh fruit and vegetables because they have great food value; they energize you.

- Lose weight to become healthy, not to become skinny. Being skinny can be just as unhealthy as being obese.
- Read this booklet to the end.
- Shop for the items listed here so you'll be ready to begin on your start date.

It can be stressful to go down the aisles of the grocery store and see all the choices available. Temptation to buy unhealthy food is everywhere. This diet is designed to limit your choices, which eases this stress. Go to the store with your shopping list in hand. Don't peruse the aisles. Go directly to those items you need and then exit the store, leaving temptation behind.

Although it did not happen to me, prepare yourself for a temporary plateau in your weight loss. This is common and it will pass. You may not even notice it if you weigh yourself only once per month.

Make your start date the first day of the month. That way, you can weigh yourself at the first of every month and see real progress. Avoid weighing yourself more often because weight can easily vary based on the day and on the time of day. When you weigh often, it feels like you are not making progress. Give yourself a break and only weigh in once per month.

The first month on this diet may be difficult. If you find yourself getting too hungry between meals, drink more water and eat as many carrot sticks, celery sticks, and clear broth as you want.

For me, with each successive month, it became easier and easier to adhere to this diet completely.

Remind yourself that this is not a quick fix. This is a long term plan to get the body you want. Sticking with it *will* bring the results you desire.

Okay. Once you have prepared yourself, you are ready to begin this diet in earnest.

Basic Daily Menu

Breakfast   Breakfast protein drink

Lunch   Black beans and salsa with a glass of vegetable juice and take two Vita Lea tablets

Before dinner Metamucil (plus two Osteomatrix supplements if you need more than 1,744 mg of calcium per day) up to an hour before dinner

Dinner   One apple, one orange, and a Premier Protein drink

Snacks   Otter Pops popsicles - one per day*

Drinks   No limit of water and two 16-oz Iced Tea with Stevia sweetener

These are the basics. You'll need to read on to learn how to shop for and prepare each item. Don't skip meals. You need the nutrition.

*Instead of the Otter Pop, you may substitute one of the following:
   1 peach
   2 carrots
   ¾ cup sliced strawberries
   1 cup asparagus
   1 cup of broccoli

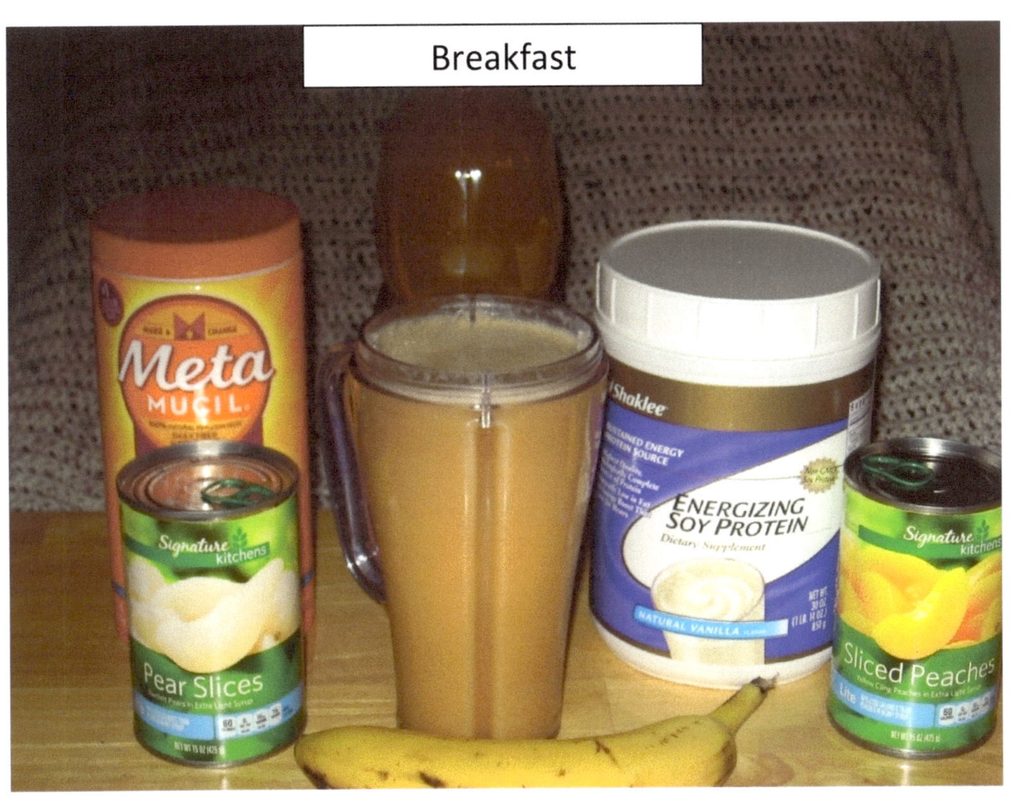
Meta
MUCIL
Signature
kitchens
Pear Slices
Shaklee
ENERGIZING
SOY PROTEIN
Dietary Supplement
NATURAL VANILLA
Signature
kitchens
Sliced Peaches
Lite

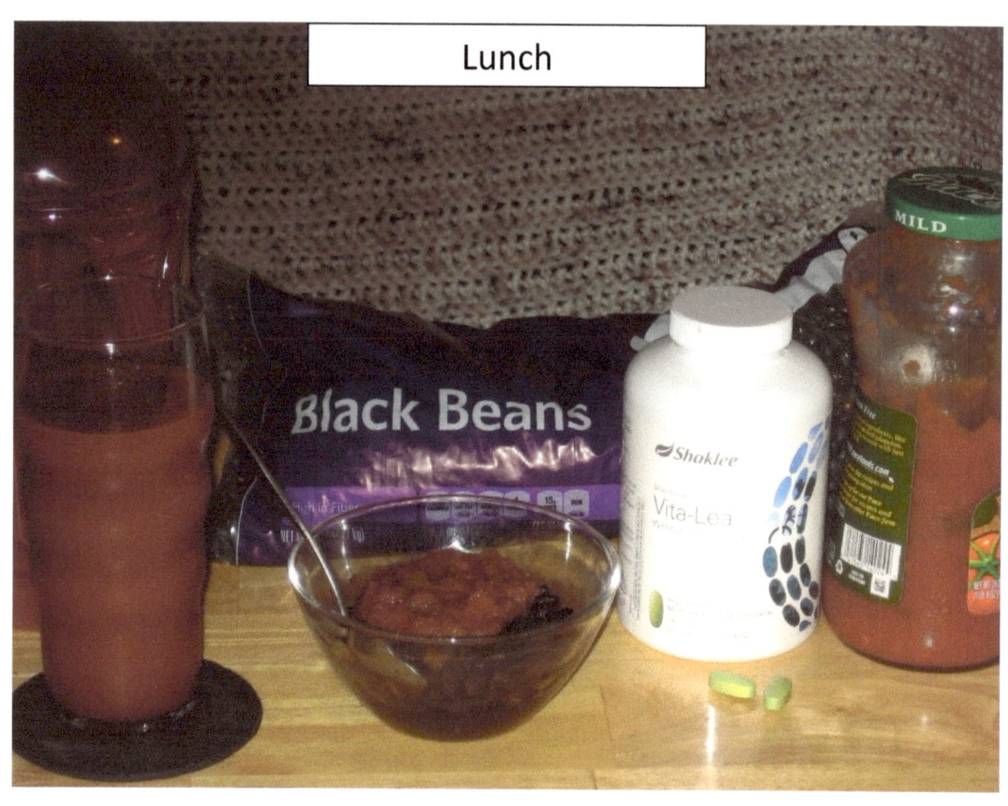
Black Beans
Shaklee
Vita-Lea
MILD

Dinner

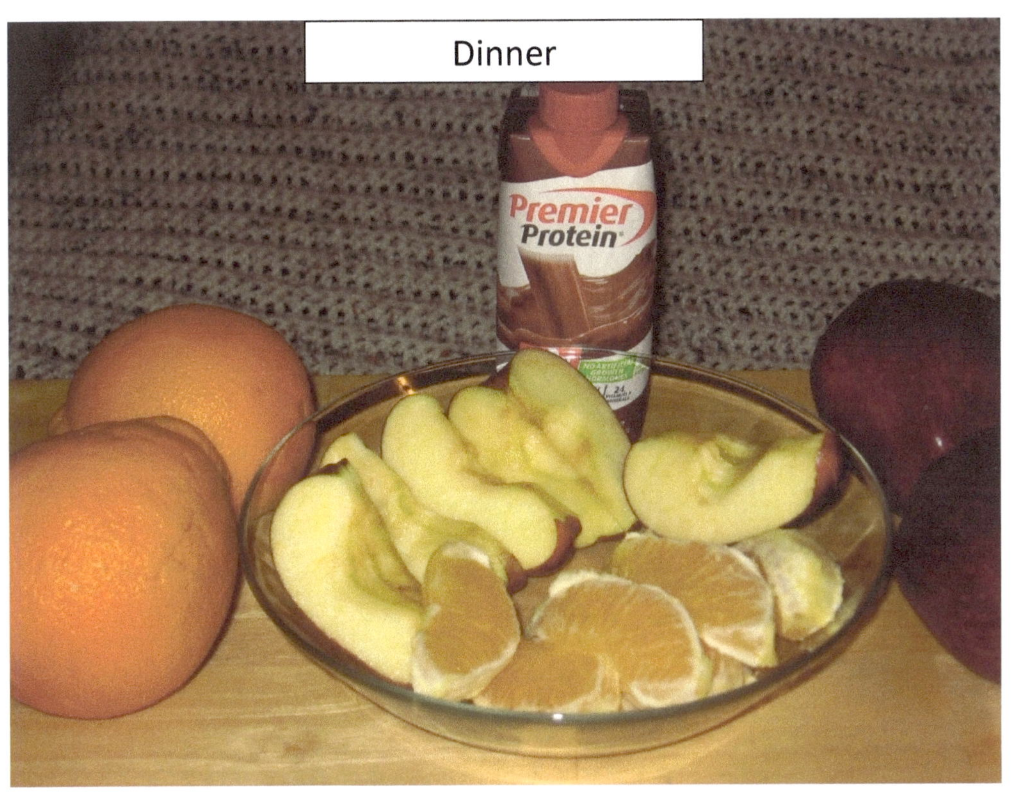

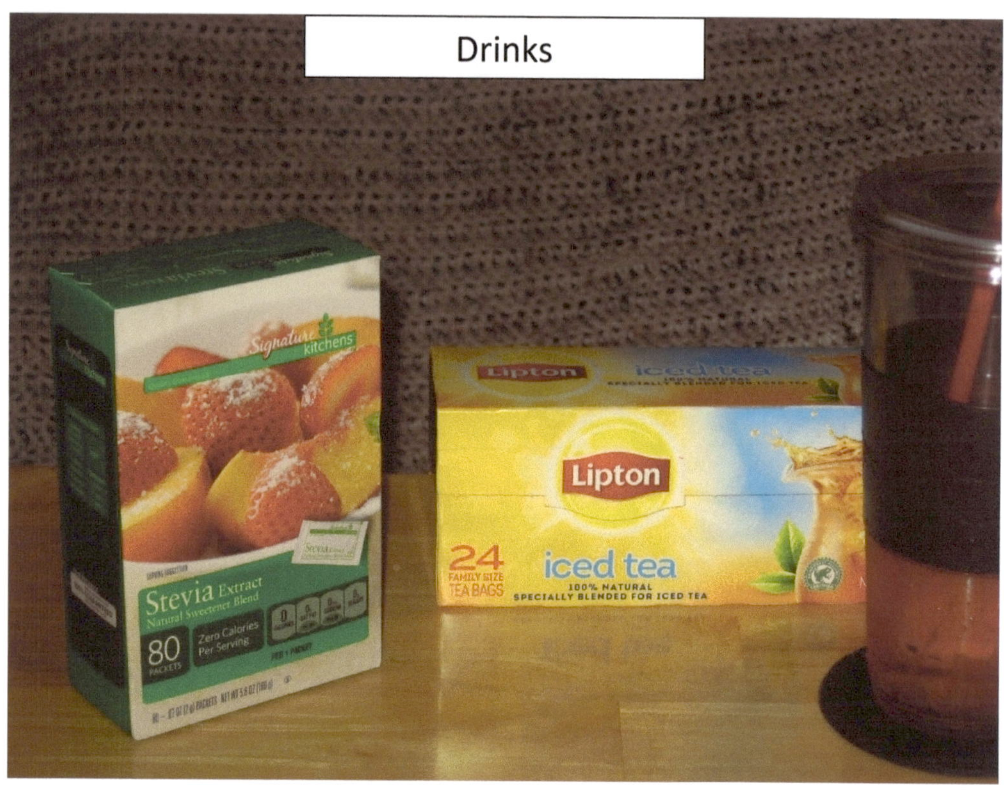
Signature
kitchens
Stevia Extract
Natural Sweetener Blend
80
PACKETS
Zero Calories
Per Serving
Lipton
iced tea
Lipton
24
FAMILY SIZE
TEA BAGS
iced tea
100% NATURAL
SPECIALLY BLENDED FOR ICED TEA

SHOPPING LIST DETAILS

Shaklee: Find your local distributor or go on the Shaklee.com website to order the following items. You'll save money on shipping if you order all of these items at the same time because there is a minimum shipping charge.

Keep in mind that the Shaklee Energizing Soy Protein container will last approximately one month, while the other supplements will each last several months.

- Shaklee Vita Lea multi vitamin multi mineral supplements. You can order with or without iron. Most women of child-bearing age order it with iron. Most women past menopause order without iron. Most men order without iron. Your doctor can help you decide which is more appropriate for you.

  These are natural, high-quality supplements in a form that can be easily digested. I don't recommend any other brand of supplement as quality differs substantially. You will take two Vita Lea tablets with your lunch each day. By the way, two Vita Lea tablets provide 500 mg of calcium.

- Shaklee Osteomatrix dietary supplement is for those who need more than 1,744 mg of calcium. Two caplets provide 500 mg of calcium, 600 IU of vitamin D3, and other nutrients that aid in the absorption of calcium.

Take these with your Metamucil drink before dinner if you need the extra calcium.

This diet is designed to provide approximately 1,744 mg of calcium per day and 800 IU of vitamin D3 without Osteomatrix.

A personal experience: I discovered that when I consume dairy products, I get calcium deposits at the base of my fingers. They can cause pain especially when grasping a steering wheel. When I take Shaklee calcium, in Vita Lea or Osteomatrix, these deposits go away. A friend of mine had the same experience. I'm not guaranteeing that everyone who takes Shaklee calcium will have this experience; just that we have.

According to www.muschealth.com, you can absorb 500 mg of calcium at a time. This is why you separate the times calcium is taken: breakfast drink (Energizing Soy Protein), lunch (Vita Lea), and with or after dinner (Premier Protein).

- Shaklee Energizing Soy Protein is a soy-based protein powder supplement. The vanilla flavor is best for this drink. You add three tablespoons of this protein powder to your breakfast drink. There is no meat in this diet so it is important to supplement your protein intake. Three tablespoons of Shaklee Energizing Soy Protein contains 500 mg of calcium.

My sister experiences hormonal symptoms (such as anxiety and a quick temper) with soy-based products. Mix your breakfast protein drink as instructed for two weeks; then have your doctor test your hormone levels to see if they need to be adjusted.

Note: Many women have hormone imbalances that require diagnosis and treatment, regardless of their diet. See your doctor and have him or her give you a blood test and, if necessary, prescribe appropriate corrective hormones to get you back in balance.

If you cannot tolerate a soy-based protein, take your Shaklee Energizing Soy Protein container to a health food store. Ask for a plant-based protein powder that is as high in quality as Shaklee's, has no more than 110 calories per serving, and at least fourteen grams of protein per serving.

I have priced them in a health food store and found that Shaklee protein, including shipping costs, to be approximately the same price as the available substitutes.

This diet has been designed to provide 59 grams of protein per day, of which, 14 grams comes from this breakfast drink if using Shaklee Energizing Soy Protein.

Costco:

- Premier Protein drinks: This is where I purchase the Premier Protein drinks you have with your dinner (or after dinner as a snack). As of 2017, you can buy 18 drinks per carton for $24.99 at Costco. I have found this product in other grocery stores but they often charge $24.99 for only 12 drinks. Premier Protein drinks contain 30 grams of protein for only 160 calories per 11 ounce drink box. The chocolate flavor tastes great! This drink contains 500 mg of calcium.

- Otter Pops: Costco is also a good place to buy Otter Pops popsicles. They are made of fruit juice and contain only forty calories per pop, according to their label. You are allowed one of these per day. I find that they satisfy my craving for sweets. They are not essential to this diet.

  You may substitute another snack for these pops; just be sure your substitute does not exceed forty calories per day. Suggestions for substitutes are listed elsewhere in this booklet.

Pharmacy:

- Metamucil: A pharmacy is the best place to purchase your Metamucil 4 in 1 Multi Health Fiber. Usually, this product costs less at a pharmacy than in grocery stores. I like the orange smooth flavor.

Place one tablespoon of Metamucil in your breakfast drink in the morning. Before dinner, place one tablespoon of Metamucil in at least eight ounces of water and stir well.

Grocery Store:

- Fruit Juice: This is for your breakfast protein drink. Choose whatever juice you like; just make sure it contains 100% of recommended vitamin C and 110 or less calories per eight ounces of juice. Before you use this juice in your protein drink, mix it half and half with water.

  For your morning breakfast drink, pour sixteen ounces of this mixture into the blender before adding the Metamucil, canned fruit or other fruit, and Shaklee Energizing Soy Protein.

- Canned Fruit: This is also for your breakfast protein drink. Buy any brand you like of canned peaches and canned pears, sixty calories per serving, fruit halves or slices. Purchase the low sugar variety. Remember, the serving size on the can is less than the amount you will use in your breakfast drink. It may read 60 calories per serving but it is 105 calories for a half-can serving used here.

Place half the contents of one can of either peaches or pears into the blender for your breakfast protein drink. Canned pears are the basis of the RDA notes above and contain 3.5 grams of fiber. Canned peaches contain no fiber.

Instead of the canned fruit, you may substitute any fruit serving that contains 105 or fewer calories. For example, according to www.chiquitabananas.com, one medium banana contains 110 calories and is a great source of potassium, 3 grams of fiber, and 1 gram of protein. One cup of strawberries is only 48 calories. One cup of blueberries is 82 calories.

Get creative!

- Iced Tea: I prefer Lipton Iced Tea box of 24 family size tea bags. Place one bag in a large pitcher and fill with cold water. It will brew in a few hours. Don't add any sweetener to the pitcher.

Fill a 16-ounce glass with iced tea and add one packet of Stevia sweetener (1/2 teaspoon). You can have two of these drinks per day. They are calorie-free.

- Stevia Extract: This is a non-calorie sweetener. It comes in ½ teaspoon packets and is available in most grocery stores near the sugar. Add one packet to 16 ounces of iced tea.

You may add less Stevia, depending on how sweet you like your iced tea.

Store some Stevia packets in your purse or wallet. When you go out for a meal, order unsweetened ice tea and add your own Stevia sweetener.

- Dried Black Beans: Each quarter cup of dried beans makes one half cup of prepared beans and contains only 70 calories per serving, provides 9 grams of protein, and 15 grams of fiber which is 60% of recommended fiber intake. This calorie count is listed on the nutrition label on the bag of dried beans. You will eat a half cup of prepared beans in your lunch with salsa mixed into them.

To cook approximately one week of prepared beans, place two cups of dried beans in a large sauce pan filled with water up to two inches from the rim of pan. Place in the refrigerator to soak overnight.

The next day, cover with cold water up to one inch or so below rim of pan. Bring to a boil; then turn down heat and simmer for two hours. When turning the heat down, place a lid on top, ajar, so that there is a one-inch gap, and leave the lid on until beans are done. The water may condense on the lid and drip. It may boil over a little. Add water occasionally to keep the beans covered in water.

When the two hours are over, take the pan off the burner and let cool for about one hour. Then place cooled prepared beans in a large bowl or container with the liquid covering them, so they don't dry out in the refrigerator.

Each day for lunch, you will scoop out ½ cup of prepared beans into a small bowl and heat in the microwave for 2.5 minutes. Remove from microwave and mix two heaping tablespoons of salsa into the beans.

Tip: An uncovered bowl of prepared black beans makes a mess in the microwave. Purchase a round dome microwave cover and place over the beans while heating them. Then just rinse out the cover after use.

Note: when I looked up the calorie count online of this portion of black beans, it showed a much higher number than 70 calories. The package of dried black beans showed only 70 calories. This is why you buy dried beans and cook them yourself.

- Salsa: Use a salsa that has only 10 calories per two-tablespoon serving and 230 mg or less of sodium. I like the flavor and texture it adds to the beans. Place two heaping tablespoons of salsa on the prepared hot black beans and mix in.

- Vegetable juice. Drink a 16-ounce serving with your lunch. Don't dilute this juice with water. Make sure the vegetable juice is one that has the following nutrients per eight-ounce serving: maximum of 50 calories, 900 mg or 26% RDA for potassium, 2 grams of dietary fiber, 2 grams of protein, vitamin A 40% of RDA, 120% of vitamin C, 2% of calcium, 2% of iron, and no more than 140 mg of sodium.

- Fresh apples and oranges - eat one of each for your dinner. I like to core and cut up the apple in wedges, leaving on the peel, and I peel and section the orange before sitting down to dinner.

The RDA percentages and calorie counts I noted assume you are eating a large Red Delicious apple with the peel on and a medium sized Naval orange, peeled. This fruit provides 33% of the RDA for fiber.

Shopping List Short Version

Shaklee   Vita Lea (with or without iron), Osteomatrix (if you need it), and Energizing Soy Protein vanilla flavor

Costco   Premier Protein drinks and Otter Pops

Pharmacy   Metamucil 4 in 1 Multi Health Fiber

Grocery

- Peaches and Pears, 15-ounce cans, low sugar variety (or substitutes as noted)
- Fruit Juice - 100% of vitamin C (with calories as noted previously)
- Lipton Iced Tea box of 24 family size bags
- Stevia Extract either packets or loose
- Dried Black Beans
- Salsa (with nutrients and calories as noted previously)
- Vegetable Juice (with nutrients and calories as noted previously)
- Apples, large
- Oranges, medium
- Any snack substitutions you choose for Otter Pops (at 40 calories each)

DAILY MENU DETAILS

Breakfast - 370 calories

Shaklee protein drink: Mix well in blender: 16 ounces of fruit drink mixture, one tablespoon of Metamucil, half of the contents of a 15-ounce can of peaches or pears (or preferred substitution), and three tablespoons Shaklee Energizing Soy Protein powder.

Drinks - zero calories

Two 16-ounce iced teas each with one packet (1/2 teaspoon) of Stevia sweetener. Drink lots of water.

Lunch - 180 calories

Half cup prepared black beans, heated 2.5 minutes in microwave. Top with two heaping tablespoons of salsa and mix in beans. Drink 16 ounces of vegetable juice. (Take two Vita Lea tablets with this meal).

Snack - 40 calories

Otter Pops maximum one per day or one of the other 40-calorie substitutes

Before Dinner - 45 calories

Mix one tablespoon of Metamucil into at least eight ounces of cold water and stir well. (If you need additional calcium, take two Osteomatrix tablets with this drink). I drink this up to one hour before dinner.

Dinner - 345 calories

One apple, one orange, and one Premier Protein drink

Note: Usually I find that I am satisfied after eating the apple and the orange. If so, I drink my Premier Protein drink a little later in the evening. The chocolate flavor tastes like I'm having a dessert

Okay, now make a commitment to yourself, complete your preparation, and get started on this diet to **Lose 40 Pounds in 5 Months Without Exercise**.

After You Lose the Weight

After you have lost all the weight you wanted to, don't return to your old ways of eating. That didn't work for you, remember?

Don't celebrate your weight loss by buying a bag of potato chips or cookies. If you want to keep this weight off for life, you need to permanently change the way you eat and how you relate to food.

You don't want to be one of those people who lose weight and then gain it all back again, sometimes gaining more than you weighed when you began.

It has now become your habit to eat less and eat better. You don't want to break these new habits; you want continue to enjoy the benefits of them.

Through these months on this diet plan, you learned to eat less and to eat until you are satisfied, not until you are full. You learned to eat only what you planned to eat. You learned that you could do without a lot of foods you used to consume. You can continue to do that and continue to enjoy your new weight for the rest of your life.

It took your commitment to prepare for this diet. It took commitment to stay on this diet. Now, it takes a real commitment to stay healthy and slim for the rest of your life, but you can do it.

You have been living with a 1,000 calorie diet for many months. If you don't want to lose any more weight, add calories to your diet. Continue to use this diet as your base calories and nutrition, and then add from there.

Your optimum calories per day to maintain your weight will differ with your gender, health, and level of activity. Ask your doctor what your maintenance calorie count should be. Then add only that number of calories to your diet each day.

Gone are the days of sodas and bags of potato chips and packages of cookies. You no longer live like that. You want to keep looking good and feeling good about yourself. This is your new life.

While adding calories to this diet, start by adding fruit and vegetables. If you like, add small portions of fish and lean meats without skin or fat on them. Grill meats in the oven so you don't have to add oil while cooking them. Also, grilling will allow the fat in the meat to drain away. Add spices to your meat for flavor. Go online and look up the calorie content of each item you add to your meals.

Sure, you can have a slice of cake at the party, but keep in mind that it will cost you approximately 250 calories that day. If your maintenance calories are 1,500 per day, then you still have 250 more calories you can eat in addition to the diet plan in this booklet.

When you go out for a meal, you can order what you usually order, but only eat half of it. Get used to leaving food on your plate when you eat out. It's okay to leave it! On the day after you eat out, you may want to eat only what you would have eaten while you were on this diet.

It's a matter of attitude. Instead of looking at all the things you don't eat, instead, think of the food besides this diet that you can add to reach your maintenance calorie level each day. You are adding to your diet, not depriving yourself.

Continue to weigh in at the first of every month. This is crucial. If you gained any weight that month, return to the diet until you are back to your desired weight. Then, go back to adding calories to maintain your optimum weight level.

If you exercise now, you will be able to add more calories to your maintenance meal plan. You'll probably feel like exercising now because you feel better about yourself.

Depending on how much weight you lost, you may have excess skin covering your newly slimmed down body. Give your skin at least one year to adjust to your new body weight. After that, only you and your doctor can decide if you want to do something more to rid yourself of excess skin.

Remember, this is the new you, your new life. If your old weight was holding you back in any way, enjoy your new freedom.

Look in the mirror and enjoy your new look. There is no such thing as a perfect body. Make friends with that person in the mirror. Congratulate her or him for the accomplishment you attained. Stand up straight and proud. Cry out, "I did it!"

If you can afford it, make the effort to go shopping for new clothes instead of wearing the old ones that are now baggy. Even thrift shop or consignment shop clothes will do. You may enjoy trying on clothes now. Don't be afraid to look good and feel good about it.

Do something with other people. You will feel more confident now, so try out your new ego. Give yourself a chance to experience feeling better around others. Take a class, go to the library or bookstore, join a club, volunteer, go out dancing, and invite someone to share these things with you. Be proud of the new you.

You earned this new weight and new life.

Enjoy!